An Anxiety Story

By Drew Linsalata

An Anxiety Story

ISBN: 978-1-7346164-2-2

Edited by Hilary Jastram

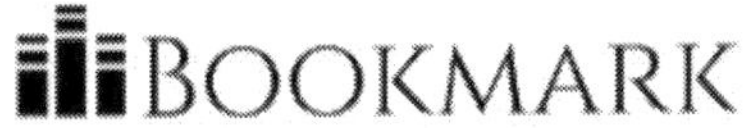

An Anxiety Story

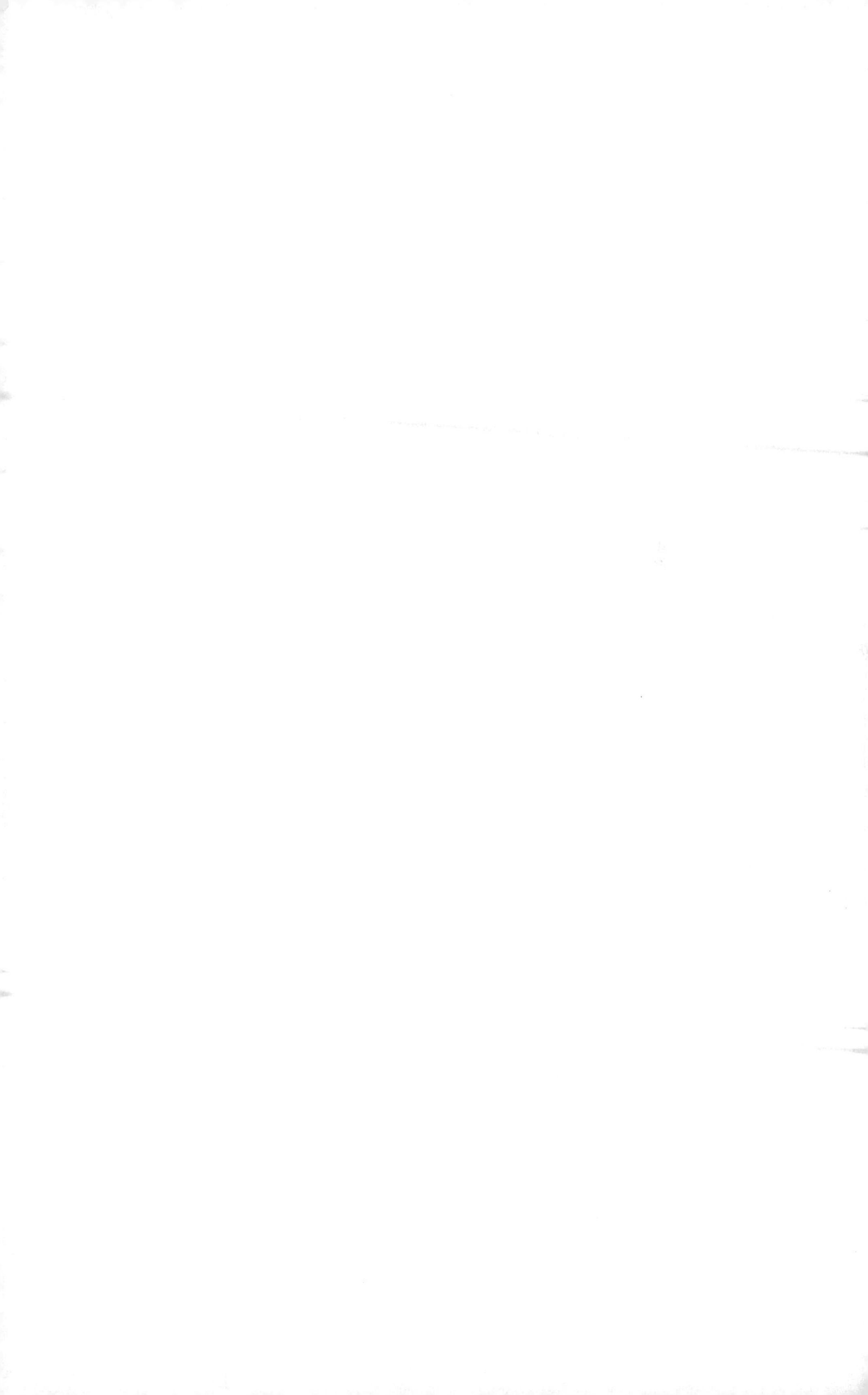

Resources

Facebook Group and Instagram Links:
theanxioustruth.com/links

Podcasts, Videos, Resources on Panic and Anxiety:
theanxioustruth.com

70,000-word Comprehensive Guide:
theanxioustruth.com/bookone

Table of Contents

Introduction

What is this book?

I was you.

This book is the story of my journey through anxiety, panic disorder, and agoraphobia. It is the story of how I solved these problems and went from an anxious train wreck to a full, productive, happy life. I have told this story before. Twice on video and once as a guest on a friend's podcast. When you're making a YouTube video or recording a 20-minute podcast, you have to leave out a bunch of stuff that people want to hear. This demands to be said in writing, so that is what I will do. I'm going to tell the story informally and conversationally as if you and I were sitting over a cup of coffee. I am hopeful that it will resonate with you.

But before I go on, let me take a short detour.

Since launching my podcast, *The Anxious Truth* in 2014, I have been asked to write a book at least once every week. I did, but this is not that book.

That book is a 70,000-word comprehensive guide. It walks the reader through an understanding of the real nature of anxiety and panic. It explains how someone can wind up anxious, afraid, and lost. It details a strategy for getting out of that horrible situation. Finally, it details how to create an anxiety recovery plan, then how to execute it. I'm quite proud of that book. It is the culmination of many years of personal experience. I based that book on research and feedback from real anxiety sufferers at all levels. I've put no less than 2500 hours into this project over 5-10 years. This includes writing, talking into microphones and cameras, and interacting with people like you. People who simply want to get their lives back. As of this writing (January 2020), that book is about to enter the editing and publishing stages. You can find more information about that book at theanxioustruth.com/book-one.

Why did I write THIS book?

I'm asked all the time if I am fully recovered from my anxiety disorders.

The answer is that I am! One hundred percent. Anxiety and panic do not impact my life now and haven't for many years.

When it came time to write the book everyone has been asking for, I knew I would have to include the full story of my journey and recovery. You can't tell someone to do things you haven't done yourself. It is important to be honest and up-front about the path I took. I want to tell the good, the bad, and everything in between. One of the things that made my podcast so popular over the last five years is the fact that I have lived through this problem myself. The things I say, the topics I cover, and the advice I give are all rooted in real experience. My listeners appreciate that, and I am grateful for the support they've given me. I owe them, and you, as a reader, the respect of telling my story before asking you to spend any money on anything else I write.

When it came time to publish my primary book, I was confronted with the nuts and bolts of the publishing process. I've always struggled with the idea of taking money for any of my words. I've accepted exactly ZERO dollars for anything I've done on this topic up to this point. So the idea of spending $7000 or more to publish a book was not sitting well with me. That was going to drive the price of the book up, and I don't want to do that. A few author friends of mine advised me that I could likely do it myself. Since this is not a business for me, and I don't have my financial future riding on the project, I thought that was worth a shot.

I needed to go through the layout, design, and publishing process and learn about that. Thus, I decided I would take the introduction to the book–the story I am about to tell–and spin it into a free Kindle book. You get the story and my background. I get to learn the publishing process, and in the end, I don't have to spend a fortune to get the "big book" out there. And I can keep the price down as a result. It is my hope that everyone wins this way.

So, why did I write this book? Because the story needs to be told regardless. Writing it as a standalone book benefits everyone associated with the whole crazy affair. I love it when a good plan comes together, don't you?

Is there more?

Yes, there is more. If you downloaded this hoping to see the entire book you've been asking for, don't freak out. The big book–the actual recovery guide–will follow this release within two or three months (as of January 2020). Everything you need to know about that book, me, the podcast, my YouTube channel, and all my social media channels is at theanxioustruth.com/links. If you haven't already, pop on over, follow me on social, and let's get to know each other. I love being able to interact with listeners, readers, and new friends in general, so I look forward to seeing you.

OK, that's enough of the introductory stuff. Let's get to the nitty-gritty.

CHAPTER 1

1986:
What Is Going On Here?

It's 1986.

My sophomore year of college, and I'm about 20 years old. I was home on Long Island, New York for spring break, in the house I grew up in. Everything was going great. I was studying architecture and getting very good grades. I had a ton of great friends and a most excellent girlfriend. I was even making good money as an intern for a well-known Long Island company during my summer vacations. The future was looking pretty bright.

Up to that point in my life, I was bulletproof. I never got nervous. I feared nothing. I was a high achiever in several areas of life without ever worrying for a second about anything. While others freaked out over exams, I didn't give them a second thought and aced them. My friends were nervous and afraid of musical auditions. I didn't practice, didn't care, and made it all the way to the all-state level on the French Horn.

I was actually playing several brass instruments at a high level. Nothing bothered me; nothing rattled me, and by all indications, that pattern was going to continue forever.

What could go wrong?

I'll tell you what could go wrong. My very first panic attack. An experience that would change my life, that I will never forget, and that led to the book you are reading right now. It was unexpected, unexplained, and terrifying. I could never have imagined the impact it would have on the next 20-plus years of my life. I promise I will not spend 400 pages describing every one of the panic attacks I've ever had. This one, though...this one is going to be explained in detail. I remember it well. So, I want to write it all down, and for you to understand that I know what it feels like all too well.

I was hanging out in my bedroom with the radio on, reading a book feeling fine. I had no indication of what was about to happen.

All the sensations and thoughts you know and hate rushed over me. I had never experienced anything like that before. It was horrifying.

First came the depersonalization. I was outside myself, experiencing myself in a jarring and disturbing way. Like I wasn't real. That by itself was enough to send me over the edge. My heart started pounding. I was alternating between sweating and freezing. I was shaking. I was breathing like I was running an Olympic relay. My vision and balance went into the trash.

Next came the derealization. Not only was I not real, but now NOTHING was real. My body was in a total state of panic. I didn't feel real; the world didn't feel real, and I was convinced that what I was experiencing was the precursor to death. I truly thought I was going to die. As I sat bolt upright on my bed, "Sultans of Swing" by Dire Straits was playing on the radio. It was late, and everyone else was asleep. I've always been a night owl, even back then, so I was alone in this state. I could have gone to wake my mother, but I thought, *what's the point? This is what it feels like when you die, so why make her watch it?*

I thought that. I believed that. I did not understand what was happening, and I interpreted it as the onset of certain death. I sat for a while. It was at least long enough for the song to end because I remember getting up and trying to walk to the bathroom down the hall. When I did that, the song on the radio was "Kyrie" by Mister Mister. You may not be old enough to know the tune, but it includes some words that you hear in a Catholic Mass (Kyrie Eleison). When you are sure that you are dying, and an 80's pop band is singing "Lord have Mercy," that doesn't help the situation.

Writing this is making me laugh a bit. It's been almost 34 years now, and I still remember the songs on the radio that night.

Convinced I was going to die and terrified, I trembled my way down the hall to the bathroom. I resorted to the "splash water on the face" trick. This had no effect, which made things worse. Even in that terrified state of panic and dissociation, I knew from a logical standpoint that water does not prevent death. Still, I moved on to gulping water from the bathroom sink, using my hand as a makeshift cup. I do not know why I did that. I was running on pure survival instinct at that point. As you would expect, it did nothing. I sat on the floor in the bathroom with my back against the wall. I remember how cold the tiles felt, but it was good because it was something I could actually feel with some certainty. At this point, I had been in that state for 10 minutes or so. The shaking was so intense. I don't shake. I never had before. But I was shaking so hard that that by itself was enough to fuel panic.

My next move was back to my bedroom. I sat on the bed. Then I got up. Then I paced. Then I sat back down. Then I jumped up and paced again. My heart was pounding in my chest, and it felt so hard to breathe. I was so disoriented and off-balance. Oddly, I did not think I was having a heart attack. I knew I was afraid, but I concluded that I was afraid because when you die, you are afraid. It all seemed so logical to me. I'm guessing that I spent a few minutes doing the stand-up/sit down/pace around the room routine. Nothing was changing. I don't think I was trying to make it stop. I was listening in on it, trying to pick up signs as to what was going on. I was watching it and waiting for the end (death) to come. I was now 15 minutes or so into it, and still, I was alive.

I remember thinking that if I could get myself into the living room and into the big blue recliner chair we had, that somehow that would be a good thing. So that's what I did. The house was dark, and for some reason, I thought that I should not shine any bright lights into my eyes. I slowly worked my way to that chair in the dark. I sat in it but didn't recline. It was also a rocker, so that's what I did. I rocked in the big blue recliner, waiting for death to arrive. Again, it did not. In retrospect, death, by not showing up, was leaving me clues that I should have picked up on. I did not. I wish I had. It would have saved much suffering later on, but I will reveal that part of the story later. At this point, I was roughly 20 minutes into the first panic attack of my life. I thought it might be time to wake my mother. I got up out of the big blue recliner and turned on a table lamp. Then I almost knocked it over, because at that moment I wasn't exactly the picture of coordination. Rather than go get my mother, I decided to sit in the big blue chair again. This time I reclined it. I remember thinking that I was getting tired.

I remember wondering how I could feel tired and terrified at the same time. That seemed odd, but I also interpreted it as additional danger. Tired was bad because if it led to sleep, I assumed I would not wake up ever again. There was no way I was going to be closing my eyes any time soon.

I laid in the big blue recliner chair, shaking, afraid, confused, and certain that I was done for at the age of 20. I remember suddenly starting to feel a little better. At that moment, I was able to consider the possibility that I was not going to die that night. I recall realizing that I no longer felt unreal. I felt like me again. Everything else still felt very strange and a bit off, but I felt real again. My heart was still beating quickly, but it didn't feel like it was pounding as much. I was less afraid but more tired. As I sat in the big blue recliner, starting to feel better little by little, my mother came out of her bedroom. She had heard the little table lamp mishap and gotten out of bed. She was surprised to find me sitting in the living room at that late hour. In one of the oddest moments of my life, she asked me if everything was OK.

I replied, "Yup. All good."

I cannot explain why I said that. It was clearly not "all good," yet that was my response. I think I did not want to jinx myself. I was feeling better and calming down, and I didn't want to talk about what had happened for fear that it would keep going. She walked back into her bedroom, and I was alone again. I sat for a few minutes longer, then got up and walked back to my bedroom. I didn't bother to turn out the light in the living room. When I sat on my bed, the world no longer looked strange to me. My heart wasn't racing. I was still shaking, but not as hard. I was feeling better, but still unstable and quite afraid. I decided to lay down but was not going to turn my light out. Fear will do that to you. It will make you not want to be in the dark.

The song on the radio at that moment was "Owner of A Lonely Heart" by Yes. I reached over and turned down the volume. I did not want total silence, but I didn't want to hear the music anymore either. I felt so exhausted–like I wanted to sleep for a year, but I was still afraid to actually fall asleep. I tried to lay there and breathe, but it was then that I made a big mistake.

Deep breaths, right?

Wrong. Within about a minute, I had started to hyperventilate. I got that unreal feeling again, and the wheels fell off. I won't go into detail because this little story is already long enough, but I jolted back out of bed. My heart was back to a million miles an hour, and the whole ordeal started again. It was less intense the second time, but still terrifying. The next two hours or so were spent riding waves of panic, with brief crashes in between. I try not to be dramatic when I talk about these things, but that was, without a doubt, one of the top three worst nights of my life. I would not wish that experience on anyone. If you're reading this book or listening to my podcasts, I'm guessing you know exactly what I mean.

Ultimately, it ended. I finally calmed down and fell asleep at about 3 AM that morning. I was so exhausted that my body had no other choice but to rest. So, it did. And I was thankful.

The Aftermath - A Long Slide Down A Steep Slope

The next morning when I woke up, everything was different. I was no longer bulletproof. I was rattled and, for the first time in my life, afraid.

What was I afraid of?

Easy. I was afraid of repeating that experience. Plain and simple. I would have given anything to ensure that it was never going to return. I didn't know what it was or what caused it. But I was totally terrified that it was going to happen to me again. This may sound familiar to you.

I won't detail every day of the next six months of my life, but I was a textbook case of progressing and advancing panic disorder. I was home for a few more days before returning to college, and they were not good days because I was a nervous wreck. After a single panic attack, I walked around the house, checking my pulse and trying to breathe deeply. I was totally on guard for whatever sensation might indicate that it was happening again.

Of course, it happened again. I had a few more attacks at home, still with no idea at all what they were, or even what they were called. Each time, I became more afraid of the next time. I managed to get back to school with my girlfriend. The rest of the semester was a blur of fear, constant anxiety, and recurring panic attacks. I developed an unhealthy "safe person" reliance on my girlfriend. There were numerous frantic trips to the university health services, and I was always convinced I was dying. At least the nurses on duty could give what was ailing me a name. They told me I was having panic attacks and that I was fine. Of particular note was the university health services psychiatrist. In my one and only session with him, he taught me to "take deep breaths" when it happened. The very next day, I was in my girlfriend's red Datsun speeding toward the infirmary because I was in a panic. Again. But this was no ordinary panic. This time my hands and feet locked up like claws. My face went totally numb. The good doctor had taught me how to hyperventilate to the ultimate degree. So fun!

I did get to have one session with my girlfriend's abnormal psychology professor, who was a very kind man. He gave me a tape with a progressive muscle relaxation exercise he had recorded. He spoke to me for about an hour about how young adults sometimes have existential crises. They realize they are no longer children, and that death is real, and then they freak out. Bless him. He tried. I am grateful for the concern he showed in that short time. That tape got all kinds of playtime on my Sony Walkman (yes, I am older than you). As soothing as his voice was, I had no idea how to use progressive muscle relaxation, and my predicament got worse and worse.

Amazingly, that semester I managed a perfect 4.0-grade point average. Another thing I will never be able to explain. Who slides into total panic disorder, begins to develop agoraphobia and monophobia, and aces every class at the same time?

This guy. Go figure.

Back home for the summer, I decided that I should see my family doctor. As another curious side note, it turns out my doctor was quite addicted to cocaine, but that's not the point. The doctor examined me and did blood tests. He scared the crap out of me by having his office call me back in for the results. During those four days of terror, before I could see him again, I assumed I had some dreaded disease. It turns out that I waited four agonizing days to find out that I might have a minor liver thing that you don't even do anything about. *Couldn't tell me that over the phone, could you?*

The doctor told me that I was experiencing "free-floating anxiety" (his exact words). He gave me a prescription for an antihistamine. Atarax. I still remember the name. It was supposed to make me drowsy. I was not a fan of taking pills, and throwing an antihistamine at this problem was like throwing a dodgeball at Superman. It bounced right off as expected.

My panic attacks and anxiety troubles continued to grow. I worked my summer job at the large defense contracting company where my mother also worked. It was a good gig, in my area of study, and paid well. The problem was that it was getting harder and harder for me to go there. I was OK in the car with my mother, or with my girlfriend, but not alone. I experienced panic in the car, which naturally led me not to want to be on the road by myself. I would not get on the highway and took side roads everywhere on every reluctant drive. At work, I experienced panic attacks several times each day. Each time they hit, I retreated to the men's room, and that was becoming untenable.

As luck would have it, the company was large enough and old fashioned enough to have a company doctor on staff, along with a real nurse. Her name was Marylin. One day rather than darting into the men's room, I walked into the health office. I asked

Marylin if I could sit there for a few minutes and explained what was happening to me. She was lovely. She sat with me and talked to me about it, and was the first person who really knew what it was. She spoke to me intelligently about what was going on. I would go to see her when the panic hit, and Marylin would sit with me patiently, trying to explain what I was feeling and why. She had a pretty decent understanding of the whole thing. After about a week of that, she gave me the name of a local psychologist and strongly suggested that I go see him. Marylin–the company nurse at that large defense contracting company on Long Island–was the first person I encountered on this journey who taught me how to help myself with my problem. She was my first teacher.

Thank you, Marylin. I'm sure you are no longer with us, but you mattered to me. A little of what you did for me lives on today in this thing that I do.

Enter Claire Weekes

The psychologist that Marylin told me could help, actually did. But not in the way you might think. I had exactly two sessions with him. In the first session, I explained what was going on. He told me that Marylin had given him some advance information, then informed me that I likely had panic disorder. He also said the word "agoraphobia" and was dead-on correct. He didn't care about my symptoms or what I was afraid of. None of that mattered to him. He didn't need me to tell him anymore because he just understood. This was my first glimpse of what so many of you have heard me talk about for five years. About 40 minutes into the session, he left the room for a minute. When he returned, he had a book in his hand.

Hope And Help For Your Nerves[1] [1]The author was Dr. Claire Weekes.

It was a small book. The cover was boring. Not much to it. He gave me the book, told me to read it, and said it would explain most of what was going on. I made an appointment to see him the following week and went home, having no idea what had just happened.

When I got home that night, I started reading. And I know this is not a good writing style, but...

Oh. My. God.

Claire Weekes was writing about ME! She knew everything I felt. She described everything I was experiencing. She knew what it was. I could not read fast enough. I am not lying when I tell you that it was a

---

[1] Weekes, Claire. *Hope and Help for Your Nerves*. New York: Penguin, 1990.

damn-near spiritual experience. I devoured the entire book that night and didn't get to sleep until 4 AM. I will admit that I called in sick to work the next day to read it again.

To have it all explained to me the way Dr. Weekes did, changed everything.

Now it had a name.

Now it had a description.

The mystery was gone. I knew what to do.

Bulletproof was back.

I know that sounds like insanity, but when I put that book down, I knew it was game over for my panic disorder. I felt so good the next day. Better than I had in many months. Like a weight had been lifted. Not anxious, not afraid, and not on guard. I was in the driver's seat again. It was awesome.

The next day, it happened. As expected, good feelings alone do not get the job done. I was back at work. All-day long, I could feel anxiety and fear creeping back in. By the time the end of the day rolled around, I was right on the edge of panic and was silent the whole way home trying to chill out as my mother drove. When we got home, I sat in the passenger seat. My mother asked if I was OK. I told her to leave me alone. She went inside, but I sat there, knowing that the rubber was about to hit the road. The book told me that I was supposed to accept panic when it happened. I was supposed to float through it. Do nothing. Don't react. Let it all happen.

Give me good information that I can act on, and I am going to do something with it. That is exactly what I did. I sank back in the seat of my mother's Ford Escort and let go. I had full acceptance of whatever was going to happen and accepted it without resistance.

If it was going to kill me, it was going to kill me. I wasn't going to try to stop it.

The panic rose up inside me and went over the top. Cue full-throttle panic and fear. It was one of the bravest moments of my life as I put my trust in an Australian doctor and the book she had written at least 15 years earlier. I went limp, did my best to breathe, and resigned to be terrified until I wasn't. Make no mistake; it was incredibly difficult to do. My eyes were closed the whole time. My body was in full reaction mode, and my brain was screaming at me to jump out of the car and run into the house to get help. But I did none of that. I just sat there and faced my anxiety attack directly and let it get me.

The whole thing was over in less than 10 minutes!

Do you know the moment where a panic attack starts to subside? That moment was the victory moment. When I felt it lessen, I was transformed into some kind of goddamn superhero. No kidding. At that moment, I knew I had slain the dragon. The war was over. *The book worked. I did it!*

That moment, on the driveway, in that little silver car, was the beginning of the end for my panic and anxiety. I know this sounds completely ridiculous, but within a few weeks, after a few more episodes, just like that, it went away. Not completely. That took a few months as I recall, but for the most part, the game was over. I no longer experienced or anticipated panic. My agoraphobic tendencies lifted, and I no longer needed my "safe people." Life returned to normal.

That six months or so of my life had been a real struggle, but it ended happily, and I was no worse for the wear.

Or so I thought.

See me again in about ten years.

Next stop…1996.

CHAPTER 2

1996:
Its Baaaaack!

In 1996 Bill Clinton was president.

The first internet dot com boom was underway. Everyone was wondering what was going to happen at midnight on December 31, 1999. Oh, and the Macarena. There was that, too.

The other thing that happened in 1996 was that the freakin wheels fell off on me again. Everything was going great. I was in the middle of that dot com boom, selling internet access to Macintosh users when Apple was about two weeks from bankruptcy. It was a good niche--almost like selling based on religion. I was living on a beach, had the coolest office ever in a 110-year old converted factory, and was having panic attacks again on a regular basis.

The previous ten years had been pretty much free of anxiety and panic. It had popped up here and there for a few minutes but was nothing I can really remember.

Slowly, little by little, it crept up on me again. I remember first noticing it, thinking that it was that old thing again, and figuring that it was nothing. If I just ignored it, it would go away. It did at first. So, I'd have an anxious day here and there. That turned into an anxious few days now and then. Then I experienced my first panic attack in ten years. The anxiety had been more and more impactful for a few days, and it all boiled over into full panic while in the car with my sister. I don't even remember what we were doing that day, but I remember feeling really anxious. I was pretty much doing everything wrong the entire time I was in the middle of it. Bracing. Fighting. Trying to talk myself down. What's odd is that I experienced that panic attack while driving on the Sunken Meadow Parkway (bonus points if you're from Long Island and know what that is), doing 70 MPH. My sister in the passenger seat had no idea what was happening. Inside I was a total wreck, but on the surface, I wasn't showing any signs. That wasn't by design, and it wasn't an accomplishment. I was fighting it the whole time, pretty much ignoring what I had learned ten years earlier.

After dropping my sister off at her place, I had to get home. Like I'd stepped back into the 1930s, I took local roads the entire way. This is ridiculous for anyone that has ever had to drive from the south shore of Long Island to the north shore. It takes WAY longer on the local roads than on the parkway, but I did not want to get back on the parkway. While that initial panic attack passed after a while, I was still very anxious, and to be brutally honest; I was afraid again.

The drive home was difficult. I stopped several times to get out of the car. I got myself a bottle of water. I intentionally altered my route to drive closer to a friend's house "just in case." I had to stop to put fuel in the car but was so anxious and increasingly desperate to get home that I only pumped a few gallons of gas. Just enough to get me to my house. I couldn't stand there while the entire fuel tank filled. When I got home, I was exhausted, shaken, and already worried about what the next day would bring. The wheels were quickly falling off one by one.

The next few days were shaky at best. The final straw was the panic attack I experienced driving home from my office a few nights later. The beach community I was living in was isolated from the main part of the Island. It was a slow drive across a narrow road surrounded by water before the road turned into a heavily wooded area. And nobody was ever on the road with you. It's still Long Island, and the isolation isn't nearly what many of you in truly rural areas experience. Despite that, I felt entirely alone and out of the reach of help during that 15-minute drive home. About two miles from my house was a firehouse. The fire department serving my community was all volunteer, and quite small. As I was in a full panic heading toward home, I had the windows rolled down, the wind screaming in my ears, and the radio turned up to an insane level. All I wanted to do was get to that firehouse to be "saved." When I arrived, it was dark. Not a car in the parking lot. Only a sad little blue light next to the front door. I sat in the parking lot, pounding on my steering wheel, beside myself. With no other option, I pointed the car in the direction of home and finished the last two miles. It may as well have been 100 miles given my state at that moment. It took forever. I'm sure you understand what I'm saying.

That was it. In the span of roughly two weeks, ignoring everything I had learned in 1986, and doing everything wrong, I was squarely in the grips of panic disorder again.

The only explanation I can come up with for this was that my experience in 1986 was a real anomaly. In all the time I have been writing and speaking on this topic, and interacting with anxiety sufferers, I have yet to encounter someone who went from anxious mess to what looked to be fully recovered as quickly as I did that summer when I was 20 years old. It was too fast. I didn't get a chance to really learn the core concepts through experience and repetition. I've come to believe that if I had struggled more and been forced to really practice the art and skill of surrendering to panic and anxiety, this second go-around would likely not have happened. It's quite odd that it did, especially since I still owned that Claire Weekes book. What I will never understand is how I never thought to take out the book and read it again. That was just stupidity on my part. Maybe I had forgotten that I had it. Who knows? But for whatever reason, I let panic take hold again, and things went downhill rapidly.

Within about two months, I became agoraphobic. I did not want to leave my house. When my business demanded that I be in the office, or when I had no choice but to go see a client, I would just endure it. I was bracing and fighting and trying my best to hold it all together. "White knuckling" my way through life. Whenever I could stay home, I did. I was in a constant state of inward focus and examination, always scanning for the next signs of panic. Always anxious. Always afraid at some level. Eventually, I was spending 90 percent of my time at my house. I remember the day my business partner came up to the house with his wife. We sat and talked about what was going on. I had to tell him that I knew it was insane, but that I was afraid to leave the house. Anyone who knows me personally knows that this was one of the most difficult things I've ever had to say. We made arrangements for me to work from home. I owned the damn company and couldn't go there. Failure is never an option in my life, but in those days, I was failing often and in spectacular fashion.

The more I fought it, the more battles I lost.

Depression began to set in. I had not experienced depression before, so that was new to me. I don't often speak about depression because I don't feel qualified to do so. I will tell you, however, that I would not wish that feeling on any human being ever. I did not want to get out of bed. I did not want to shower or get dressed. Being hungry became a nightmare because I didn't want to think about what to eat. That was just too much to handle. Nothing had meaning. Nothing had context. It was like the color had been flushed out of the world completely. I lost the ability to feel any kind of connection to anyone important to me. It was totally de-humanizing. I never hit the point of being a danger to myself, but I felt like a shell of me. While anxiety and panic were bad; for me, depression was far worse.

So there I was, afraid, lost, and severely depressed, living in a very small world. At times the combination of panic and depression was unbearable. I recall two emergency trips to the doctor because I could simply not take it anymore. The first trip was to a doctor on call. He was covering for my regular doctor one evening and agreed to see me. To his credit, he tried to explain that I could be helped, but I wasn't listening. He did mention therapy, but I couldn't hear it. I wanted an immediate fix. He was not my usual doctor, who would be back and available in just two days, so he did not want to do anything too major. He wrote me a prescription for a benzo. Exactly four pills. This was a conservative doctor without a doubt. I do not even recall his name, but he deserves credit for not jumping into the deep end of the pool with his prescription pad, even though he knew I wanted immediate relief. He was a kind man and compassionate.

When I went to see my regular family doctor two days later, I heard the words that now make me cringe.

"You have a chemical imbalance."

You don't need to hear me rail on about neurochemistry and pharmaceutical marketing, so I'm not going to go that in-depth. Keep reading, and you'll see that I did, in fact, spend nine years taking an antidepressant after this doctor visit. I try hard not to have regrets in my life, but this is about as close as I can get to one. Back to the story.

I have never been one to take medication. I rarely take an aspirin if I have a headache. I have to be genuinely sick to take something. When my doctor said he wanted to give me a couple of medications, I resisted. In fairness to him, I was making unreasonable demands. I wanted immediate relief from my suffering, but I also did not want to take any pills. So, he was never going to be able to satisfy me. He responded to my reluctance with a line I am guessing that many people may have heard.

"If you were diabetic, you'd take insulin, right?"

I pressed him on side effects and potential pitfalls. He minimized my concerns and planned on giving me a "gentle" antidepressant. It was going to be fine. I just had to wait 7-10 days for it to start working, and I wasn't allowed to stop taking it without talking to him. While I was waiting, he gave me a prescription for thirty Ativan (lorazepam) pills. Thirty. To get me through 7-10 days. He said nothing about the addictive nature of benzodiazepines. He didn't advise me to use it only when needed. It was supposed to calm me down while the antidepressant "built up in my system."

At that point, if there was a way for me to just sleep for ten days, I'd have taken it, anything to escape what I was feeling. I agreed to try the medication. So, I left, got two prescriptions filled, and went home.

On about day six, I opened my eyes in the morning. The sun was up. I felt different. I didn't feel empty.

It was like my depression had lifted. I do not mind telling you that I cried a little. I felt almost human again. I was still quite anxious and feeling unstable; but the depression was markedly lower, and I was grateful at a level that I can't describe even to this day. As opposed to antidepressants as I am now, at that moment, I was a believer.

I still experienced anxiety for the next week or so. However, even though I couldn't judge it very well, it felt like it was getting better.

One afternoon I was on the phone with my office. Things got a bit heated because of an issue we were having with a vendor. I felt my anxiety rising. All the signs were there. It was coming again. Panic was knocking. Loudly. Then...it stopped. The best way I can describe it was as a "short circuit." Like someone had lit a fire, but before it could grow, someone else threw a bucket of water on it. It fizzled, then went away. I sat at my dining room table and cried again.

Over the next week or so, everything changed. My depression was gone. My anxiety was gone. The fear was gone. I went outside again. The color was back in my world. I began popping into the office here and there, staying for an hour or so at a time. I remember sitting in the office, staring out the window for a bit. Everyone knew that I wasn't fully back yet, but they were nonetheless happy to see me. That was a real boost. Over the next couple of weeks, my visits to the office become longer and more frequent. I got stronger and stronger. Then it was time to go back to work, so I did. I was a little nervous that day, but it was a good nervous, mixed with a bit of excitement and a bunch of optimism. The nightmare was over.

Oh, and I had taken exactly zero Ativan. So I had that going for me.

As life returned to normal, and I got back into the swing of running things and being me again, I was ready to declare this a happy ending. Through the miracle of modern medicine, I had my life back, and it was good.

Until it wasn't.

Next stop...2005.

CHAPTER 3

2005:
The Antidepressant Withdrawal Nightmare

By 2005 so much had changed.

I lost grandparents. My two daughters were born. I gained 100 pounds. I nearly destroyed a business, lost a home and a family. I alienated all my friends and taught my kids that Daddy didn't care. Good times.

Remember how amazing my antidepressant was? Turns out...not so much.

It took away my depression and my anxiety. It took away my panic attacks. What it also took away were all my emotions, my good judgment, and my ability to give a damn about anything. I wasn't depressed or afraid. I wasn't anything. I lived without a connection to my family and friends. I made completely unexplainable choices when it came to money and how to spend my time. I drove my business to the brink of extinction. I went into debt. I ate whatever I wanted to and as much as I wanted to. I didn't move. I locked myself away behind computer screens. It was not good by any measure.

When my grandparents passed, I didn't shed a tear. I felt nothing. When my daughters were born, I went through the motions. I never got happy or sad. I never got excited. I never felt anything–anger, sometimes, but even that was not common. This was clearly not a normal state for a human being. I was truly a different person than I was before I started taking that medication.

Physically, I became very unhealthy. As I noted, I gained 100 pounds. *One hundred pounds*. I'm not a little person, but I don't care how wide your shoulders are, very few humans should weigh 310 pounds. I couldn't walk up my driveway without getting short of breath. I was sweating all the time, regardless of the weather. My blood pressure was high. My cholesterol was high. When tested, I was showing early signs of type 2 diabetes. It was quite the party.

Here's the most insidious part of the whole ordeal. I KNEW that it was all wrong. I knew that my mother was right when she begged me to do something to stop the slide. I knew that I was not supposed to shove four slices of pizza in my mouth for dinner, then a fifth as a snack two hours later. I knew that I was supposed to be more engaged with my family. I knew that it was wrong not to pay the taxes on my house. I was aware that spending money that I didn't have was a bad idea. I knew all this, but for some reason, it just didn't matter. I could not grasp the gravity of the situation no matter what consequences I was facing. Anyone who knew me before or after the medication is absolutely astounded to hear that this was me between 1996 and 2005. I assure you, it was. I still don't believe it, and I *lived* it.

To make matters worse, four different doctors in nine years didn't give it a second thought. Every one of them continued to tell me that I just had a chemical imbalance that required me to take meds for the rest of my life. When I complained that something was different about me, they all dismissed it. That's not a side effect of Paxil, I was told. Gotcha. Not a side effect.

But again, I wasn't anxious or depressed. So...mission accomplished! Yay!

(Since I can't put an emoji in a book, I will ask you to imagine the eye roll emoji here. Thanks.)

One day I came home from what passed for work, plopped myself on my bed with my laptop like I always did, and got busy doing nothing productive. You know, a typical night. My girls were about five and three at the time. They were in the 5-year old's room playing. Then they walked out and headed for the living room with a bunch of toys in tow as little kids are prone to do. They had something planned.

My 3-year-old stopped in the doorway of the bedroom and asked if I would come to see what they were doing. I didn't look up from my laptop. I just said, "OK, pumpkin. I'll be right there."

She stood in the doorway of my room, waiting.

Her older sister finally came back to get her. She grabbed her hand and took her toward the living room. The words my oldest daughter said in that moment will bring me to the edge of tears until the day I die. Oh, and those words also both changed and saved my life.

"Come on, let's go. He's not coming. He just says that."

My daughter said that. She told her little sister that. She was right.

If there is a single moment in my life around which everything revolves, it is that moment. For years, I heard nothing. I took no advice. I listened to nothing that would help me. I did nothing to help myself. I ignored it all and kept rolling toward disaster. Then my daughter casually reached out and slid her finger right through all the armor and indifference. *She quite literally poked my soul, then walked away to play with her little sister, oblivious to the impact she had.*

Allow me to be a dad for just a second here:

"Bunny, I know that at some point, you will read this. When you do, please know that if my words help just one person in this world, they have you to thank. At the tender age of five, you changed everything for me. Thank you, and I love you."

OK, back to it.

I slammed my laptop shut. For the first time in many, many years, I cried.

At that moment, in the dark, at 310 pounds, flat broke and broken by many measures, I resolved that this would not continue. If it hadn't been 7 PM at that time, I'd have gone directly to my doctor right then and there to tell him that I was done with the medication. I left a message with his answering service and arrived there promptly without an appointment at 9 AM the next morning. I got myself in the door, in front of the doc, and explained the deal. He was confused and not too convinced that this was a good move, but he said OK, then gave me the typical tapering advice that everyone gets. I went a bit slower for good measure, then took my last dose of Paxil in September of 2005. My taper lasted roughly 6-7 weeks after nine years on the medication. That was not OK, as I was soon to find out.

The next six months or so was a nightmare of uncontrollable and unpredictable emotions. There were relentless waves of fear, crushing depression, and panic attacks. There were also obsessive non-stop nihilistic thoughts focused on death, dying, and the futility of existence. You may think I am being dramatic or exaggerating. I assure you I am not. It was absolutely crippling. Every thought, sensation, emotion, and sensory input was magnified, distorted, and weaponized. I had no control over any of it. I knew anxiety, panic, fear, and depression, but this was a whole new variation on that theme.

As you would expect, I turned to my doctor for help. He kept telling me that this was my chemical imbalance showing and that I needed to go back on the medication. I clearly remember the day I sat on his exam table while he said that for the fifth or sixth time. I stood up, took a step toward him, and told him in no uncertain terms that I would sooner die than do that. I absolutely meant it, too. After what my daughter said, there was no way I was going back there. I suppose the look on my face was enough to tell him that I was serious. He sat me back down and pulled up a stool.

We talked for a good 10 minutes or so. He said he would support me, only on the condition that I came to see him EVERY DAY. That's right. Every day. He also insisted on giving me a prescription for Xanax and made me promise that I would use it when I was near the breaking point and needed some relief. He was clearly concerned about me in a big way, but still said he'd work with me as best he could. He did admit that this was new territory for him, which I appreciated. We shook hands, and I left there with him in my corner. He is still my doctor. I respect him for doing what he did. He went above and beyond for me, and I will be eternally grateful for that.

By the way, he gave me 90 Xanax pills. I threw away 89 of them 18 months later. Yes, I am a stubborn mofo.

I was managing antidepressant discontinuation (withdrawal) while also merging my business with a local telephone company. That was incredibly difficult to do. It was like admitting defeat, but without the medication clouding my judgment, I could do what I knew was the right thing. It did mean that I had to get up in the morning, go to an office, and keep regular hours. That was terrifying to me. I did it every morning in an elaborate ritual of binaural beats playing in my earphones, magnesium supplements, green tea (decaf, of course), and deep breathing. None of that really did anything, but I hoped it would, so I did it anyway. I had virtually no ability to recall information from memory. As I was trembling quite often, I would sit in my office with my headphones on, listening to Ron & Fez and Opie & Anthony on satellite radio and checking my blood sugar periodically. To have something strong to smell, I burned candles. I was splitting my time between actual work and obsessively reading the PaxilProgress website.

Let's talk about that for a bit. PaxilProgress was a web forum dedicated to helping people going through what I was going through. There were so many of us there, all sharing information and experiences, trying to feel better, and trying to help each other. That website no longer exists, but at the time, it was a literal lifeline for me. I made friends there that are still my friends. I learned how to help people there. I am grateful that PaxilProgress existed. To Laurie Yorke, my friend, and the woman responsible for that site, thank you from the bottom of my heart.

Slowly, purely based on the passage of time, things improved. I had no magic tricks to make it happen. No herbs. No supplements. No attempts to micro-manage my brain chemistry or "fix" things. Just time. That's what it took. Over time, my brain found its way again. Between the day of my last dose and the time that I achieved some level of stability, I was able to enjoy some really interesting activities. Here's a partial list for your entertainment:

- ✓ *Jumping up and down like a frog when I thought I couldn't feel my legs.*
- ✓ *Carrying a paper bag with me at all times in case I might hyperventilate.*
- ✓ *Not eating Chinese food because I thought it caused a panic attack.*
- ✓ *Checking my blood sugar because I was convinced it was crashing, and I was going to die.*
- ✓ *Constantly checking my pulse to see how fast it was.*
- ✓ *Constantly poking my chest because I was so terrified of my own heart-beat.*
- ✓ *Crying uncontrollably for two days at the series finale of Six Feet Under.*

- ✓ *Crying uncontrollably for an hour over a toilet paper commercial on TV.*
- ✓ *Not being able to look at any bright lights.*
- ✓ *Getting angry at my kids for using the word "dead" in normal conversation. I had to circle back a year or so later and explain that it was OK.*
- ✓ *Frantically throwing my stuff in my bag at 4:59 PM every day so that I wouldn't accidentally be the last person in the office. Being alone was BAD.*
- ✓ *Going to my doctor's office every day for two months. Then every other day. Then twice a week for a while. Then weekly until I was out of the*

woods. (I got to know the staff very well.)

The list is much longer, but I won't bore you. You get the idea. Over time, my emotions smoothed out. I wasn't experiencing those random crying jags anymore. Of course, then the issue was experiencing every emotion as panic, but that also got better over time. The periods of crushing depression and nihilism also faded. When I realized that I hadn't felt that for two weeks or so, *that* was a good day. The sensitivity to light improved, which was a big deal. I was tired of walking around with my hand over my eyes like I was looking into an eclipse.

One night in the fall of 2006, I came home and wound up just petting the dog on the living room floor for ten minutes or so. Ten minutes of not thinking, not feeling, not scanning, and not being on guard. Just petting the dog. It was amazing.

One moment that I really want to acknowledge came the day my doctor told me I didn't have to come see him anymore. He shook my hand. He told me that he would have never believed that what I experienced was real had he not witnessed me go through it. I thanked him for sticking with me. It was a learning experience for us both. Walking out knowing that I didn't have to return was a big deal.

That experience was horrific. The worst of it lasted every bit of eight months or so. I would not wish it on my worst enemy, but to be totally honest, I would do it all again today if I knew I would wind up where I am right now. The experience taught me things. I learned the art of helping other people from my friends at PaxilProgress. I learned a HUGE lesson in seeing acceptance for what it was on any given day. I discovered how to be more patient than I ever thought I could be. I learned that there is a difference between pain and suffering. I learned that humans are amazing and adaptable and capable of astounding feats of emotional and mental strength.

I gained an appreciation for the art of letting go of anger and bitterness. That was a big hurdle. I was incredibly angry at the drug company that made Paxil and at every doctor that told me that I had a chemical imbalance. That anger was not helping me. It served as a bit of motivation for a while, but mainly it was damaging and drew my focus away from where it needed to be. Deciding to let that all go was one of the greatest eye-opening acts of my now almost-54 years on this planet. I urge you to learn this art, too. It can change your life.

I found reasons and ways to look beyond the nuts and bolts of daily life. I gained an appreciation of spirituality and the desire to make sense of our place in the universe. I read things. First, to soothe my irrational fears, then to incorporate valuable lessons into my world view. I paid attention to things I never cared about before. I learned to recognize when self-applied labels were causing problems rather than helping. Did I really need to be "Type A," an overachiever, or impatient? Above all, I learned to find the lesson in every experience, regardless of the outcome or perceived goodness or badness. This serves me well to this day.

I was righting the ship with my business and finances, engaging with my family, and heading in the right direction. I went from 310 pounds to 240 pounds with no effort whatsoever. My blood pressure went down. My cholesterol went down. I was back to being an intelligent, responsive human being with a moral and ethical compass and a sense of good judgment.

Let's recap.

Add the antidepressant; things go sideways fast.

Remove the antidepressant; things get back on track. Amazing how that worked.

At the end of 2006, I was still not perfect, but I was getting better. I was doing all kinds of good things. The one thing I was NOT doing was the work that actually needed to be done to address the issues I had ten years earlier.

There was one more recovery chapter to write.

I'll see you in about a year, in 2008.

CHAPTER 4

2008: Everything Changes

2006 ended on the upswing.

And 2007 was a pretty good year for a while. I was remodeling my house, building a deck around the pool, not overthinking how I was feeling, and enjoying being part of my family again.

As you are likely guessing, we're not quite at the happy ending just yet. There was more struggle to come. I'll get to that in a minute. In hindsight, I think I needed the first eight or nine months of 2007 to just live life again for a while. I did precisely that. It was a break for my brain and my soul. Yes, I was still living in the dreaded "acceptable bubble," but it gave me a chance to get my act together. In retrospect, I could regret not going straight into the heavy lifting of facing my fear and un-learning it, but I don't. Everything happened as it was supposed to happen. What was to come next was painful. I put everything I had into it. I approached it with a determination and tenacity that I might not have had without this little break. In the end, the first nine months of 2007 is a part of my story that I am happy to have lived.

I remember when I started to feel some of the old anxiety feelings creeping in again. They would pop up at work while I was in my office. Then they'd pop up in the car while I was driving. Sometimes they would pop up at home. I freely admit that I made the same mistake I did in 1996 when I thought to ignore them, and sometimes "run them over" was a good idea. It wasn't a good idea in 1996, and it still wasn't in 2007. Panic popped back up in various situations, and while I won't say that my slide was as deep as it was eleven years earlier, things did get progressively worse.

By the time we got to Christmas of 2007, I was neck-deep in my panic disorder again, and my agoraphobia was on the rise. For the third time in my life, I was afraid of my own body and mind. I started modifying my life to avoid those experiences that I feared and disliked so much.

This time I added Tai Chi and a half-assed attempt at meditation to the mix, thinking that my newfound respect for all things Zen would solve the problem. Not so much. While Tai Chi might look beautiful and can be calming and help with focus, thinking that it was going to banish my anxiety issues was silly. (I'd give myself an eye roll emoji here, too.)

Things progressed down the expected path. More avoidance. More fear. Less activity. You know the drill. Hell, I knew the drill by then. All too well.

If you recall, in early 2006, I had merged my company with a local phone company. It was the right move at the time, even though I hated having to do it. By early 2008, we were dismantling that deal. An unfortunate health catastrophe struck my friend who owned that company. Without him steering the ship, the business was failing. I did what I could, but the writing was on the wall. It was time to undo the merger and spin my business back out. This was a sound business decision, but it didn't help me with my anxiety issues. The first indication that this was a lousy move anxiety-wise came when I left a reasonably substantial salary increase on the table and gave it to one of the guys who worked for me. Am I generous? I'd like to think I am, but in exchange for the money, I said I would take more time off. If you believe this was a red flag, you are right. I wanted more time off not to travel the world or write the great American novel. I wanted more time off because I was struggling to go to the office every day. See the problem there? I engineered myself right into additional avoidance behavior.

De-merging the companies was easy. We were still sharing data center space and network infrastructure, which I would remain responsible for, and it was a smooth transaction. Everyone was on board. That was great because it was stress-free from a business standpoint, but again, it wasn't helpful to my health. After my last day in the office, a huge weight lifted off my shoulders. Not because I hated it there, but because I knew I didn't have to get up and go in on Monday morning. The relief was significant. If taking more time off was a red flag, this was a red flag the size of Texas, and it was on fire. Avoidance and retreat in high gear are never good, but they made up my entire life strategy at the time.

The next 6-7 months saw me go right back to being riddled with panic, and agoraphobic, and monophobic. You already know all the details from my last two go-arounds, so let me point out a few new items. I was leaving business on the floor daily because I was afraid to go to meetings with clients and potential clients. I worked from my home office every day and refused to go to my data center only three miles away.

There's only so much you can do without actually being at the business sometimes. That wasn't good. My company, at the time, was operating 24/7 (the network never sleeps), so I was in constant fear that I might have to leave the house alone and go to the office to tend to something in the middle of the night. I was afraid every day that the phone would ring, and I'd have to get in the car to go somewhere. I was barely getting the stuff done that I needed to get done.

I remember one Sunday morning particularly well. The planets had aligned against me in every way. Nobody was home at my house, so I was alone for a few hours. Not good. I was already on the edge of full panic as a result. To make matters worse, I had to spend some time reconfiguring a few long-range wireless network links. The goal was to make configuration changes, then apply them to live network elements. A mistake would mean that I would lose contact with the routers, and subsequently, parts of the network would be offline. Very bad when you are already at level eight on the anxiety scale. The idea that I might have to go out in that state to drive 20 minutes away to fix broken components was terrifying.

Side note: Let me say without being shy that I am very good at what I do. I remember an inhuman number of passwords and commands effortlessly. I have a deep understanding of the architecture of my systems, so nothing is a mystery. I also have total control over all of it. I regularly manipulate advanced networks with minimal effort and rarely, if ever, make a mistake. I know what I am doing, and I am always confident in doing it. I never worry about it…except when I did nothing but worry about it because I let myself slide headfirst into a raging anxiety disorder again.

Back to that Sunday morning. I was shaking like nobody's business. I was sweating and disoriented.

My legs were like jelly. My heart was pounding. I was at the all-you-can-eat anxiety symptom buffet and wasn't leaving any time soon. To combat this, I made myself sit at the computer in my home office, but before I could do anything, I had to get some paper. Paper. Actual paper. And a pen. I had to take almost 40 full minutes to write out every keystroke I had to type to accomplish what I needed to do. I wrote myself a key-by-key script to do this easy network reconfiguration. Then I checked it once, verified it again, and even went through it all one more time. I triple checked every password. Then I tried them by logging into the routers just to make sure. When I thought I was ready, I began my task.

I had to stop seven or eight times because I was in such a state. I had to slowly and carefully type everything that I had written on the paper, in the sequence in which I had written it. I was terrified that I had forgotten something. Not because making a mistake is scary, but because a mistake would have meant leaving the house to fix that mistake. I would do one subtask, then get up and walk around. Then do another and repeat. It took me 90 minutes to complete a task that would take me no more than five minutes to do today. When I finished, and everything worked, I walked over to my sofa and collapsed. I was exhausted and relieved but couldn't rest. I worried that I had forgotten some detail and that my phone would ring soon with a problem due to something I had missed. It was ridiculous. When I look back, I cannot believe that I was in that state, trying to live a life that way.

My daughters were learning how to ride horses around that time. The stables are only about 20 minutes from my home, but I could not take them there. I could only go if the whole family went, and even then, spent half the time off to the side with my headphones in listening to some kind of relaxation recording.

This is important to note because one day, those horses produced the final "final straw" of my life. On the day of riding lessons, the girls were naturally excited. Young girls and horses. It's a thing. Their mom got tied up when we were supposed to leave and was not going to get back out to the house in time to take them. That left...me...by myself...to drive them 20 minutes to riding lessons, wait there during the lesson, and drive home. It's a simple thing, isn't it? Dad takes his daughters to an activity they like to do. But it wasn't. We rescheduled the lesson.

That was the end. Final straw. No more. I promised myself that day that I was never going to do that again, and I resolved to do whatever I had to do to keep that promise. There was simply no way this nonsense was going to ruin my life anymore. Fool me once...but really? Fool me THREE times? I don't think so. I was about as angry as I can ever remember being, and that anger became fuel.

The winter of 2008-2009 was pretty brutal in New York. It was cold, snowy, and icy. I was neck-deep in all of it. I didn't care. In my "big book," I write extensively about recognizing what the problem is, understanding why it happens, making a plan to un-do the mess, then executing that plan. This is what I did. I already knew what it was and why it happens. I just didn't ever do the planning and execution part, and that had bitten me in the rear end at least two times. *That is NEVER going to happen again*, I told myself.

So, I sat down and wrote out a list of all the things that I feared. I ordered them from smallest to largest, and then I started facing those fears. If I was afraid of it, I did it. Relentlessly. Every day. With ZERO days off. I am not lying here. I took no days off during the execution of my recovery plan. It was easily five to six months before I allowed myself to take my foot off the accelerator and re-adjust based on my progress. Breaks are the devil in this process, so this was critical. Yes, we get tired. When we are tired, we rest. But I knew for me that most of the time, "rest" was just an excuse for avoidance, and I would have none of that in my life.

I got up every single morning, immediately got dressed, got myself ready, and went out the door to do scary things. No medication. No herbs. No supplements. No self-compassion. No self-care. Just a relentless drive INTO fear and panic every single day. I had one job: to learn how to experience anxiety, panic, and fear properly so that I would not fear them any longer. I did whatever I had to do to get the job done.

I had to teach myself how to make a morning routine, then how to execute that routine slowly, deliberately and mindfully so that I could walk out my door with anxiety at a level five instead of ten. I did that morning after morning after morning, experiencing all the symptoms and sensations and just letting them be there while I did my tasks. I never knew that brushing my teeth could be so impactful, but it was. I learned how to panic while brushing my teeth, and it mattered.

I would get dressed, sit at the kitchen table for exactly 60 seconds to reset, then get in the car and drive. My focus was on time first, then distance. I would drive in a panic for a set amount of time, then return home. I did that a few times every day. With repetition, and without fighting the panic, that length of time became easy to achieve. When that happened, I would increase the time, which would naturally trigger panic. Again, I repeated the process until that length of time became easy to handle. Next, I added distance and repeated the process again and again and again. There was fear. There was panic. There was anxiety. There was anticipation. I did it all anyway, and I did it productively.

I need to clarify that the most important thing I did through all of this was that I never retreated or avoided. Never. I didn't bail out when I would panic. I would stay in the situation, intentionally letting the panic happen. I planned my exposures and executed them regardless of how I felt. I never saw anxiety or panic as the problem. The problem was my reaction, so I worked on that tenaciously. And you need to know it's not magic. It's just how human brains work, so I leveraged that.

I knew it would work. I never doubted that it would. Thankfully I've never been bitten by the "I'm afraid I'll never get better" bug. I always knew I would get better, but only if I made myself better. Once I resolved to do that, *what I knew to be true turned out to be true*. In about 5-6 months, I went from panic at the mere thought of leaving my house, to getting in the car and driving around normally. I was back in my business. I was shopping. I was taking my kids places.

I was heading back to being a regular human. As I got better at not reacting in fear to panic and anxiety, not only when I was driving but when I was doing other tasks, everything else I wanted to do and did do got easier. I was OK, being home alone. I was OK, being at my office alone. I even went there now and then at night just because I could.

That first 5-6 months built me an "acceptable zone" where I could pretty much live 80% of life in a normal fashion. But in this game, "acceptable" is death, and I knew this. So, I kept pushing as far as it was practical to push. Progress became slower, of course, because it's hard to keep finding reasons to drive 50 or 70 miles away from home when you don't have to. I had to plan those things and schedule them, and even when I knew I didn't have to do them, I did.

It made a difference. That extra push is what truly teaches us the actual lesson we need to learn. I didn't teach myself how to take my kids to the mall; I taught myself how *not to fear how I felt* or *what I thought*. When you learn that lesson and ingrain it through repetition, the war is truly over.

I started the hard work right around January 1 of 2009. By July or so, I was firmly in my acceptable zone, and maybe 65% recovered. By the end of 2009, my acceptable zone was large enough that you really wouldn't even call it that. I'd say I was 85% recovered. That final 15% is really hard to assess. It involves the biggest, scariest challenges on your recovery "fear ladder" (I explain that in the big book).

Those are the things that you can't readily do often. They are one-off events most times. For me, that was things like going to concerts and sporting events and flying to other cities. I didn't have to do those things, and they didn't come up regularly, but when they did, I jumped at the opportunity to do them. Yes, there was some anticipatory anxiety and fear, but it was all quite doable when it was time to take those final steps.

In the end, over the following few years, I got to the point of what I would say is complete recovery. I am confident in saying that I do not have an anxiety disorder anymore and never will again. I am free from the baseless fear that dictated terms to me for far too long. Not only is the dragon dead, but I learned that it never had any actual teeth.

Why? Because I learned how to be 100 percent accepting of how I might feel, and zero percent afraid of it. Contrary to all the conventional wisdom and popular opinion, it was as simple, dry, and mechanical as that.

Some people hate it when I say that. I think there's beauty and comfort in it.

CHAPTER 5

Some Final Thoughts

Was this life-changing?

Many people tell me daily that anxiety and panic have ruined their lives.

Let me tell you this. An anxiety disorder has the potential to ruin a life. I won't pretend that's not true. But the process of recovering from an anxiety disorder can change a person in ways that you can never imagine. My experiences were not positive or happy. They were often pretty bad, and there were many of them. But in the end, the *lessons* they taught me are amazing.

I not only got the old me back, but I got a better version of me out of the process. So it's not that an anxiety disorder isn't going to make you a better person. It's that recovery from that disorder will.

This is a good time for me to acknowledge the support I had along the way. Around the time I was getting bad again in 2008, I started searching YouTube for videos about anxiety. The first person I found was a guy in Sweden who called himself JP of Diamonds. His channel is long gone. He made a series of probably 20 videos talking about having panic disorder and agoraphobia, and how he worked his way through it all. I will never get a chance to speak to him, but those videos were really motivating for me on days when I was frustrated and exhausted.

I also made a group of friends, and we shared videos back and forth. We'd do exposures on video, share them, cheer for each other, and generally support each other. If you follow the podcast or YouTube channel, you already know Billy from Anxiety United. There was also Chris, Ben, Sarah (she's been a guest on the podcast), and Emma. That little group turned into something called PanicStation, where even more awesome humans joined in. Tina, Lydia, Sabrina, Natalie, Chrissy, Sharon, and others really helped create an environment where my insane level of refusal to be defeated by anxiety was encouraged and supported. Sharing my challenges and successes with those good people helped me learn how to deliver this message. I love all of them, and I owe them all a debt of gratitude that will also never be repaid.

Sometimes I wonder why I didn't do this work in 1986. For whatever reason, I didn't really have to do it. Maybe the problem hadn't progressed far enough when I found the Claire Weekes book. Maybe my 20-year-old brain was different than my 40-year-old brain. Perhaps there is life on other planets. I don't know. What I do know is that my first run-in with anxiety and panic was just too short. It didn't teach me the real underlying lessons I needed to learn about it. I didn't get the opportunity to learn through repeated experiences with evolving outcomes that it wasn't something to fear or avoid.

I also wonder why I didn't do the work in 1996. Again, I will never really know. The book that changed everything the first time was sitting right there in my house, yet I never thought to pick it up and revisit it. How different would my life be had I done that? I likely would have never wound up on that medication. I would not have gone through the withdrawal process. I would not have gone through what I went through in 2008 and 2009. I can only imagine how different my life would be.

I am absolutely OK with how it all played out. Our lives are our lives. Every experience matters. They all teach us things. We don't exist to only slide down rainbows into pools of honey. We live to experience everything the universe can create for us to experience. Some of those things are challenging and hard. VERY hard, but those experiences become part of us. When processed in a healthy way, they make us stronger and broader and fill us with more of what I think it means to be truly human.

I do not regret any day that I have lived up to this point. I spend absolutely no time worrying about what happened or even thinking about what happened. Hell, it took me ten years to actually write it all down. In reality, I likely would not have done that if so many people hadn't asked me to do it!

I'm happy. My life has been exactly what it was supposed to be. At the risk of sounding cheesy, I'm pretty sure that every new day is the best day of my life. If I didn't think you could get to this place, too, I would not have spent all the time I've spent on this topic for many years now.

If I did it, you can do it. If I believe in you, try believing in yourself. I promise it is well worth the effort.

Before we move onto resources and the Q&A section, how about we take a look at a full chapter from the "big book"? It's all about the need to eliminate avoidance and turning INTO the fear.

What's a first book without a sneak preview of the second, right?

CHAPTER 6

Big Book Sneak Peek: Stop Avoiding— Going INTO Fear

An excerpt from my full recovery guide releasing in spring 2020.

Throughout this book, I talked about why avoiding the things you fear doesn't help you in any way. Rather than solving this problem, avoidance makes it worse. Avoidance is seeking short term-comfort, but it reinforces long-term suffering.

So, it's time to stop avoiding. It's time to start going toward your fear rather than away from it. If you've ever heard about exposure therapy, this is it. Intentionally going toward fear is the basis of exposure. In this chapter, we will talk about what it means to go directly toward your anxiety and why this will help you in the long run. If you're already imagining things you don't want to do and getting nervous at the thought of having to do them, congrats! You just took the first tiny step in the right direction.

Being intentionally afraid and uncomfortable seems like a ridiculous plan, doesn't it?

Well, aside from the fact that nobody wants to be frightened and uncomfortable, there's a reason it seems absurd to you. The faulty cognitive link between fear and danger is still trapping you. In your mind, being afraid and being unsafe are the same thing, and you've been acting accordingly. I would never tell you to do something dangerous, but right now, when you hear me say that you must go toward your fear, you're hearing me telling you to do the unthinkable. You're hearing me urging you to run toward certain death, insanity, embarrassment, or whatever else you fear will happen when you are afraid. I've had people get furious at me for even suggesting this approach because they are filtering my words through that erroneous connection between discomfort and peril. Some tell me that I am out of my mind.

These are the people who view being afraid as something you should NEVER intentionally do. I might as well be telling them to jump off the nearest 50-story building. They genuinely see it that way. Do you see it that way?

Being unwilling to even entertain this notion is a function of not accepting the error in cognition that I am describing. If you're ready to bail because the idea of going toward the things you fear seems unthinkable, I urge you to consider how often you make incorrect judgments daily.

We are wrong all the time about all kinds of things. We form opinions that turn out to be incorrect. We pre-judge. We draw faulty conclusions and make bad decisions based on incomplete or wrong information. We think we know something only to see suddenly that we never really did. Being wrong is a universal human function. If you can be wrong about your last boyfriend or girlfriend, why can't you be wrong about being in danger during a panic attack? Think about it.

So why do we have to go toward the fear? Why do this crazy thing? How will this solve your problem? To answer that, we need to look at the mechanism of learning.

Humans learn in several ways.

1. We learn by passive assimilation of information. I tell you how to scramble an egg, and you learn how to do it. You read a book about how to make scrambled eggs, and you incorporate that information into a cognitive model of egg scrambling. But while you may listen and read, you have still not scrambled that egg.

2. We learn via modeling. You can watch YouTube videos of chefs scrambling eggs. By viewing, you add to your knowledge. Your

cognitive model of what it means to scramble an egg grows and gets stronger. This cognitive model is great, but no matter how many videos you watch, that egg is still intact in your refrigerator. You haven't scrambled it yet.

3. We learn by doing. Doing equals experiential learning. You go into the kitchen armed with the knowledge you've gained from reading and watching, and you scramble your first egg. You may make a mistake or two. It may turn out badly, but then you try again, and again. After a few tries, you are enjoying a delicious scrambled egg that you made yourself.

To solve this problem of ours, we need methods 1 and 2, but the real magic is in method 3: Experiential learning. You will solve your problem by leveraging the amazing ability of your brain to turn a cognitive model into overt behavior and to refine that behavior through repetition.

We go toward the fear because we must learn through experience that while you are afraid and uncomfortable, you are not actually in danger. We do this to break that erroneous fear/danger connection that fuels your anxiety problem and keeps you stuck.

No amount of talking about it, reading about it, hearing explanations, or watching videos of people doing it will break that connection. Only DOING–learning through experience–will break it and set you free.

Sadly, this is where many people stumble. They spend a tremendous amount of time thinking about this. They read. They learn. They discuss. They, however, remain unwilling actually to DO. Thinking and learning and reading and talking is part of this process, but only the doing will matter, so you have to be OK with that idea.

You must start from these premises:

1. A mistaken link between fear and danger fuels your intense desire NOT to do this.

2. While you hate going toward your worst fears, you are not actually in any danger. You must trust that you are safe even though your brain is SCREAMING at you that you are not.

3. By doing this hard thing in the PROPER way (we'll get to that soon), you will break the mistaken link, and you will learn how NOT to be afraid of how you feel when anxious or in a state of panic.

If you're good with hanging your hat on these three premises, let's continue. Let us get a deeper understanding of what going toward the fear is all about.

It's never the thing or the place. It's always how you feel while doing the thing or going to the place.

This is critical.

If you are afraid of being in the supermarket, it is not about the supermarket at all. The supermarket is irrelevant in this equation. Your fear of the supermarket is the same fear that makes you afraid to be alone, makes you find all the hospitals around you at all times, and makes you check your pulse 200 times in a typical day. If you fear the drive-through at McDonald's because it makes you feel trapped, then you also fear driving on the highway because you can't just get off any time you want to. You fear getting involved in a conversation with an old friend after church for the same reason. McDonald's, the highway, and the friend waiting to start a conversation are all the same thing. Attack one, and you attack them all.

When we talk about going toward the fear, we talk about the fear itself, regardless of where or why it appears. If you want to be able to go to Disneyland with your family, you must learn to stand and have a conversation with your old friend after church because it's the same fear. You fear how you feel because you've linked it to danger.

In the end, it's always that, so we will attack the fear, not the specific tasks or destinations. I don't care about those. I only care about the experience of passing through fear and discomfort in the most constructive, non-reactive, non-avoidant way. If that's in the supermarket, great. If it's in your front yard, great. If it's in an airport, that's fine too. It doesn't matter.

I need you to remember this. Too many people get stuck, thinking that each task or goal is unique. They are not.

If you understand the mechanism at play, you will have a much easier time moving from goal to goal without having to re-think and "prepare" each time. After starting this journey, people often say that they're making great strides, only to ask how to tackle something new. The answer is always the same. If you've managed to get good at the supermarket, tackling your dentist appointment next month is based on the same exact mechanism and will involve the same approach. You won't have to continually ask how to do the next item on your goals list. You'll already know from having done the first few things.

Ultimately, going toward fear means:

1. Putting the brakes on your old avoidance and retreat routines. Those must be left behind.

2. Identifying the tasks, places, and situations that make you feel anxious or trigger panic.

3. Identifying your current safety rituals and behaviors so you can be prepared to drop them while going toward fear.

4. Going toward these tasks, places, and situations without engaging in those fear-driven safety behaviors and rituals. You have to learn to do these things without going into freak out mode. This is the "secret sauce" that makes the entire recipe work. I talk about this in the big book.

5. Learning how to tell the proper story about your ventures into fear and discomfort. Constructively describing those experiences to yourself and others is part of the solution to this problem.

As with many of these lessons, I'm going to ask you to take a little time to think about this. Wrap your brain around what lies ahead and what you need to do. Ask yourself if you're ready to intentionally put yourself into the situations you've been avoiding for so long. It will be unpleasant and difficult at first.

There's no way around that. It will get easier over time, though. I promise.

As you think about this, keep one important thing in mind. You will never be fully "ready" to do this. You will be afraid. You won't want to do it. That's the way it's supposed to be. That's why this works. Do not make the mistake of thinking that you must learn how not to be afraid before you start this process. You can't learn how not to be afraid until you do these things we're going to discuss. Only through the doing–the being afraid–can you lose that fear.

Get yourself ready for a leap of faith that this process will work.

First, you will leap, then you will learn. Not the other way around.

To learn more about my full recovery guide, visit my website at theanxioustruth.com/recoveryguide.

CHAPTER 7

Resources

There are plenty of resources...

And before I answer some of the more common questions that I am asked, let me share a few resources (besides this book) that are available to you.

I've also written a 70,000-word comprehensive guide to panic and anxiety issues. The guide is written for people who are anxious, afraid, confused, and lost. It will take you through understanding the problem and how you got here, understanding the solution, building a recovery plan, then executing that plan. The book is the result of many years of experience, research, and interaction with thousands of people that have the same problem that I had, and that you do now. You can find more about the book here:

theanxioustruth.com/bookone

Aside from that guide, I've spent quite a bit of time putting out a mountain of completely free information and advice about this topic over the years. You can find it all on my website.

theanxioustruth.com

Every podcast episode and video I've ever done is there. You'll find links to my Facebook group and all my social media accounts. I urge you to check it all out if you have not already done so. There is a good possibility that I've answered almost every question you can think of already in a podcast episode or video.

I'm also going to ask a favor. If you listen to my podcast, *The Anxious Truth,* and enjoy it, please take a moment to rate and review it. You may be listening via Apple Podcasts, Google, Spotify, or another platform, but regardless of where you are listening, if you can rate and review the podcast, it helps other people find the information they might need.

Also, if you downloaded this book from Amazon, iTunes Books, or Google Play, please take a moment and give it a quick rating and review. I'd really appreciate that.

Now let's get on to those questions, shall we?

CHAPTER 8

Answers To Common Questions

Finally…the Q&A!

Since I started *The Anxious Truth* podcast in 2014, I've been asked thousands of questions by thousands of good people. There is a pattern, and many questions are repeated quite often. I thought it might be helpful for me to include a few of them here, so let's get to it.

Did you take any medication?

As you can see, I did for about nine years. Given a chance, I would not do that again. When I stopped taking Paxil in 2005, that was the last anxiety-related medication I've ever used. I did all the work in 2008 and 2009 without it.

Do you ever have anxiety or panic attacks?

Once in a while, I will have an anxious day or two. I might even have a panic attack a couple of times a year. I don't care when it happens now. It's a non-impact event in my life. You'll notice that I've never said I was anxiety-free. I fixed an anxiety disorder. I did not rid myself of every shred of anxiety forever. That's not realistic. Humans experience anxiety and fear sometimes. We don't have to be afraid of that. That's the point here.

Did you have a therapist?

When I was going through antidepressant withdrawal, I did have a therapist for a while. She was a clinical social worker, and she was terrific. She was not an anxiety disorder specialist, but she let me set the agenda, offered some excellent tools along the way, and helped me clarify the direction I needed to go. I am a big fan of professional help, especially if you can find yourself a therapist that specializes in anxiety disorders and treats them with the most effective methods. When I did all my real recovery work, I did not have a therapist.

Do you recommend any natural ways to help anxiety?

What I did was all-natural. There were no side effects or chemicals involved in the work I did. Behavior isn't made in a lab. This is not a body problem. I have no recommendations on things to swallow to "help anxiety."

Isn't there a gentler, more comfortable way? This is so hard.

Yes, this is hard. Hard is not impossible, and you can do hard things. I know you can. But no. Not to my knowledge. This is what worked for me.

Did you do this all alone? Did your family help you?

I did the work I did alone and primarily in silence. That's just my way. I told everyone what I was going to do, told them just to let me do it, and assured them that leaving me alone was the best thing they could do. I promised to reach out if I needed help. That worked very well for me. I was very aware of the trap of "safe people," so I needed to make sure that I squashed all of that from the start. I also knew that talking about how I felt all the time was part of the problem, so I didn't want to keep doing that.

I think my anxiety is worse than everyone else's.

Your anxiety is no different or worse than anyone else's. It's not unique, special, or overly complicated. You are afraid of your own body and mind. This does not take away your humanity; it just points out an essential aspect of how our brains work. Embrace it and use it to your advantage. First, drop the mistaken belief that you are somehow unique or worse than everyone else.

What about diet and exercise?

I'm a fan! I am a big gym rat, and I really do try to give my body what it needs to be healthy. I enjoy being in good shape. Exercise is an excellent form of stress management. It can even be used as part of exposure therapy. However, I must say again that this is not a body problem. Be healthy. Take care of your body because it's the only one you have. But do not waste time trying to find precisely the right foods to eat or exercises to do to make this problem go away. You haven't discovered it yet for a reason, so stop looking.

Did you get (insert symptom here)?

Any symptom I might list here doesn't matter; that's why I didn't get specific. There are no special anxiety symptoms. They are all just different expressions of the same fear. So the fact that maybe you have stomach issues where I had more heart issues is irrelevant. I urge you to embrace this concept. It's part of what will set you free.

How can I talk to you?

I would love to be able to talk to everyone who wants to speak to me. It's just not practical or possible. I am not an anxiety coach or therapist, so I do not do one-on-one coaching or counseling. The best way to communicate with me is probably in my Facebook group, where I am quite active. I tend to be active on Instagram, too. You'll find links to both of those places at theanxioustruth.com/links.

Can I pay you in some way for all of this?

I am amazed at the number of people who want to pay me for telling them what I know. I never shared my story and the credible resources I found to make money, but your generosity and desire to express gratitude is very touching. If you didn't already, feel free to buy a copy of my "big book," which you will find on my website. I'm using it in part to help support mental health charities. If you'd prefer not to do that, then just make a contribution to the charity of your choice or help someone in your town who might be struggling to eat today. That would make me happy. Oh, and if you know someone else who might benefit from my seemingly endless stream of words, share the website or podcast with them. In the end, all I ask in return for the time I spend on this topic is for you to pay it forward in some way. If we all shared our experiences more freely and unselfishly, the world would be a better place.

About the Author

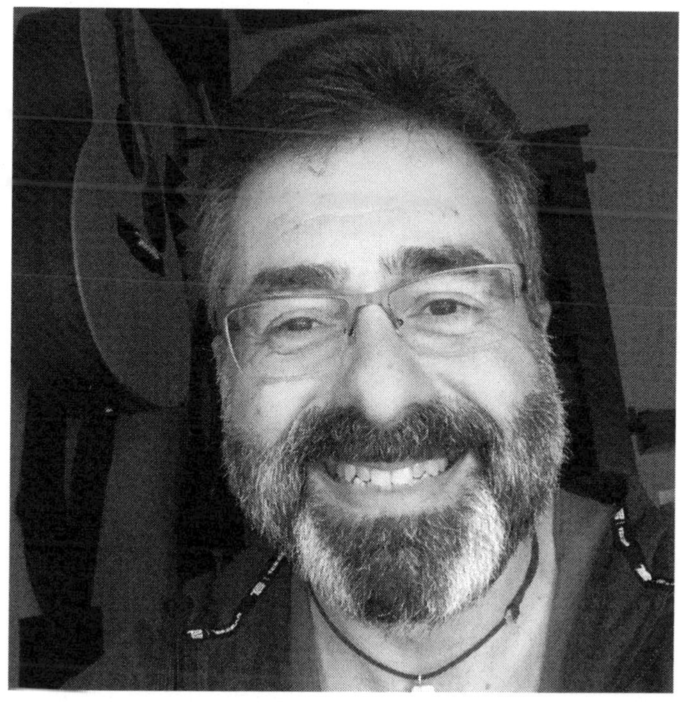

Drew is the creator and host of *The Anxious Truth*, a stunningly popular anxiety podcast that's been in full swing since 2015. With over 500,000 downloads (and growing), *The Anxious Truth* enjoys a large, vibrant and engaged social media community of amazing humans supporting, inspiring, encouraging and empowering each other to overcome anxiety and fear. Listen to a few episodes of the podcast, and you'll know right away that this isn't what you're used to hearing about anxiety.

Drew's unique, no-nonsense approach to solving the anxiety problem combines his strong, confident voice with genuine care, compassion and a desire to see others learn and succeed. You can find Drew, his podcast, and his community at theanxioustruth.com.

Having been through not one, not two, but THREE different periods of debilitating anxiety, panic, agoraphobia, and depression, Drew turned it all around in 2008.

Armed with a deep understanding of the cognitive nature of this problem, courage, and an intense desire to solve the problem once and for all, Drew rid himself of the irrational fear that fuels the disorder.

Now living a normal, happy, productive life without avoidance and retreat, Drew spends a fair amount of his time tending to his podcast, writing about anxiety disorder issues, and interacting with the large community surrounding his work.

A technology entrepreneur by day, Drew's true passion is using his own knowledge and life experience to teach and empower others as they work to solve their own anxiety and fear problems.

When he's not podcasting, writing or taking care of business, you can find Drew attempting to be a proficient guitarist or in the gym. A fan of scientific inquiry, Stoicism, Taoism, and Buddhism, Drew is also a lifelong night owl who's probably staying up too late right now.

Oh, and Drew realizes that writing about himself in the third person is a bit ridiculous, but that seems to be the way it's done in these parts, and there's nothing wrong with a bit of ridiculousness now and then!

Disclaimer

I am not a doctor. I am not a licensed therapist or counselor. This book is simply the story of how I overcame my anxiety-related problems. It was written to provide information, inspiration, understanding, and hope to the reader. I have made every effort to ensure that the information in this book was correct at press time. While this book is designed to provide accurate information in regard to the subject matter covered, I assume no responsibility for errors, inaccuracies, omissions, or any other inconsistencies herein and hereby disclaim any liability to any party for any loss, damage, or disruption caused by errors or omissions, whether such errors or omissions result from negligence, accident, or any other cause. This book is not meant as a substitute for a direct expert in the advice of medicine or mental health. If such assistance is required, the services of competent professionals should always be sought.

Made in the USA
Coppell, TX
15 May 2020

25574507R00074